The Complete Dash Diet Lunch & Dinner Cookbook

Easy And Delicious Dash Diet Lunch & Dinner Recipes

Peter Haley

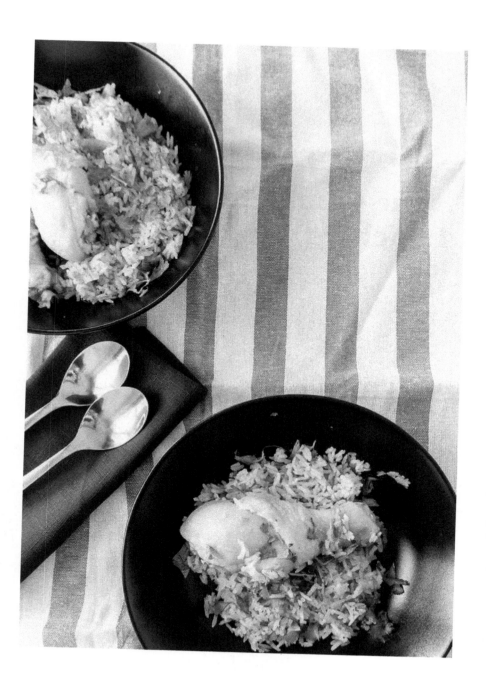

Table of contents

Buffalo Chicken Salad Wrap

Prep Time: 10 mins

Servings: 4

Cooking: 10 mins

Ingredients:

- 3-4 oz chicken breasts
- 2 whole chipotle peppers
- 1/4 cup white wine vinegar
- 1/4 cup low-calorie mayonnaise
- 2 diced stalks celery
- 2 carrots, cut into matchsticks
- 1 small yellow onion, diced (about 1/2 cup)
- 1/2 cup thinly sliced rutabaga or another root vegetable
- 4 oz spinach, cut into strips
- 2 whole-grain tortillas (12-inch diameter)

Directions:

1. Set the oven or a grill to heat at 375°F. Bake the chicken for 10 mins per side.
2. Blend chipotle peppers with mayonnaise and wine vinegar in the blender.
3. Dice the baked chicken into cubes or small chunks.
4. Mix the chipotle mixture with all the **Ingredients:** except tortillas and spinach.
5. Spread 2 oz of spinach over tortilla and scoop the stuffing on top.
6. Wrap the tortilla and cut it into the half.

Nutrition:

- Calories 300
- Fat 16.4 g
- Carbs 8.7 g
- Fiber 0.7 g
- Protein 38.5 g

Honey-Mustard Chicken

Prep Time: 10 mins

Servings: 4

Cooking: 15 mins

Ingredients:

- ¼ cup honey
- ¼ cup yellow mustard
- ¼ cup Dijon mustard
- 1 tbsp olive oil

Directions:

1. To a medium bowl, add the honey, yellow mustard, and Dijon mustard. Whisk to combine. Taste to check for flavor balance, adding more honey and mustard if necessary. Set aside.
2. In a large skillet, add the oil and chicken.
3. Cook over medium-high heat for 3 to 5 mins, then turn over and cook for an additional 3 to 5 mins. Cooking

time will vary depending on the thickness of the chicken. Chicken should be almost cooked through.

4. Add the broccoli and stir to combine, making sure the broccoli gets coated with honey mustard. Cover and cook over medium-low heat, allowing the broccoli to steam for about 3 to 5 mins or until broccoli is crisp tender and chicken is cooked through and an instant-read thermometer registers 165°F.

5. Serve immediately.

Nutrition:

- Calories 254
- Fat 8g
- Carbs 21g
- Fiber 2g
- Protein 27g

Grilled Chicken, Avocado, and Apple Salad

Prep Time: 15 mins

Servings: 4

Cooking: 8 mins

Ingredients:

- Cooking spray
- 2 tbsp olive oil
- 3 tbsp balsamic vinegar
- 4 (4-ounce) skinless, boneless chicken-breast halves
- 8 cups mixed salad greens
- 1 cup diced peeled apple
- ¾ cup avocado, peeled and pitted
- Optional: 2 tbsp freshly squeezed lime juice

Directions:

1. Preheat grill to high heat. . Apply cooking spray to the grill rack or broil the chicken in an oven-safe skillet under the broiler element for 5 to 6 mins.

2. Combine olive oil, balsamic vinegar, and lime juice in a small bowl. Place chicken on a large plate. Spoon 2 tbsp of oil mixture over the chicken, reserving the rest for the salad dressing. Turn chicken to coat and let stand for 5 mins.

3. Place chicken on grill rack. Cook for 4 mins on each side or until an instant-read thermometer registers 165°F. Remove and put on a plate. Cut crosswise into strips.

4. Arrange greens, apple, and avocado on 4 serving plates. Arrange chicken over greens. Drizzle reserved dressing over salads.

Nutrition:

- Calories 288
- Fat 16g
- Carbs 8g
- Fiber 5g
- Protein 27g

Turkey Cutlets with Herbs

Prep Time: 5 mins

Servings: 4

Cooking: 8 mins

Ingredients:

- 2 tbsp olive oil
- 2 sliced lemons
- 1 package (approx, 1 lb) turkey-breast cutlets
- ½ tsp garlic powder
- 4 cups baby spinach
- ½ cup water
- 2 tsp dried thyme

Directions:

1. In a large skillet over medium-high heat, heat the oil
2. Add about 6 lemon slices to the skillet
3. Sprinkle the turkey-breast cutlets with garlic powder and black pepper

4. Place the turkey cutlets into the skillet and cook for about 3 mins on each side until the turkey is no longer pink and is slightly browned at the edges
5. Remove from heat and divide turkey between 4 plates
6. Add the spinach to the pan along with ½ cup of water and steam, stirring frequently for about 2 mins. Remove the greens and lemons with tongs or a slotted spoon and divide between plates
7. Serve topped with dried thyme

Nutrition:

- Calories 204
- Fat 8g
- Carbs 8g
- Fiber 4g
- Protein 30g

Chicken Curry

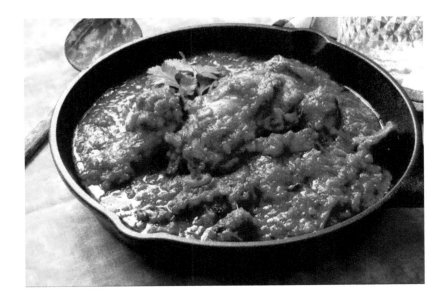

Prep Time: 5 mins

Servings: 4

Cooking: 20 mins

Ingredients:

- 3 tbsp red curry paste
- 1 lb. ground chicken

- 1 tbsp tomato paste
- 2 tsp dried oregano
- 1 cup tomato sauce
- Olive oil

Directions:

1. Heat the oil in a rice cooker
2. Add curry paste and stir
3. Place the chicken into a heated rice cooker
4. Cook until cooked thoroughly
5. Once cooked add tomato paste, and sauce.

Nutrition:

- Calories 315
- Protein 39g
- Carbs 25g
- Fat 9g

Honey-Mustard Chicken

Prep Time: 10 mins

Servings: 4

Cooking: 15 mins

Ingredients:

- ¼ cup honey
- ¼ cup yellow mustard
- ¼ cup Dijon mustard
- 1 tbsp olive oil

Directions:

1. To a medium bowl, add the honey, yellow mustard, and Dijon mustard. Whisk to combine. Taste to check for flavor balance, adding more honey and mustard if necessary. Set aside.
2. In a large skillet, add the oil and chicken.
3. Cook over medium-high heat for 3 to 5 mins, then turn over and cook for an additional 3 to 5 mins. Cooking

time will vary depending on the thickness of the chicken. Chicken should be almost cooked through.

4. Add the broccoli and stir to combine, making sure the broccoli gets coated with honey mustard. Cover and cook over medium-low heat, allowing the broccoli to steam for about 3 to 5 mins or until broccoli is crisp tender and chicken is cooked through and an instant-read thermometer registers 165°F.

5. Serve immediately.

Nutrition:

- Calories 254
- Fat 8g
- Carbs 21g
- Fiber 2g
- Protein 27g

Grilled Chicken, Avocado, and Apple Salad

Prep Time: 15 mins

Servings: 4

Cooking: 8 mins

Ingredients:

- Cooking spray
- 2 tbsp olive oil
- 3 tbsp balsamic vinegar
- 4 (4-ounce) skinless, boneless chicken-breast halves
- 8 cups mixed salad greens
- 1 cup diced peeled apple
- ¾ cup avocado, peeled and pitted
- Optional: 2 tbsp freshly squeezed lime juice

Directions:

1. Preheat grill to high heat. . Apply cooking spray to the grill rack. If you don't have a grill, broil the chicken in

an oven-safe skillet under the broiler element for 5 to 6 mins.

2. Combine olive oil, balsamic vinegar, and lime juice in a small bowl. Place chicken on a large plate. Spoon 2 tbsp of oil mixture over the chicken, reserving the rest for the salad dressing. Turn chicken to coat and let stand for 5 mins.

3. Place chicken on grill rack. Cook for 4 mins on each side or until an instant-read thermometer registers 165°F. Remove and put on a plate. Cut crosswise into strips.

4. Arrange greens, apple, and avocado on 4 serving plates. Arrange chicken over greens. Drizzle reserved dressing over salads.

Nutrition:

- Calories 288
- Fat 16g
- Carbs 8g
- Fiber 5g
- Protein 27g

Chicken and Spanish Rice

Prep Time: 10 mins

Servings: 5

Cooking: 5 mins

Ingredients:

- 1 cup onions, chopped
- 3/4 cup green peppers
- 2 tsp vegetable oil
- 1 8 oz can tomato sauce*
- 1 tsp parsley, chopped
- 1/2 tsp black pepper
- 1-1/4 tsp garlic, minced
- 5 cups cooked brown rice (cooked in unsalted water)
- 3-1/2 cups chicken breasts, cooked, skin and bone removed, and diced

Directions:

1. In a large skillet, sauté onions and green peppers in oil for 5 mins on medium heat.
2. Add tomato sauce and spices. Heat through.
3. Add cooked rice and chicken. Heat through.

Nutrition:

- Calories 428
- Fat 8 g
- Protein 35 g
- Carbs 52 g

Turkey Cutlets with Herbs

Prep Time: 5 mins

Servings: 4

Cooking: 8 mins

Ingredients:

- 2 tbsp olive oil
- 2 sliced lemons
- 1 package (approx, 1 lb) turkey-breast cutlets
- ½ tsp garlic powder
- 4 cups baby spinach
- ½ cup water
- 2 tsp dried thyme

Directions:

1. In a large skillet over medium-high heat, heat the oil
2. Add about 6 lemon slices to the skillet
3. Sprinkle the turkey-breast cutlets with garlic powder and black pepper

4. Place the turkey cutlets into the skillet and cook for about 3 mins on each side until the turkey is no longer pink and is slightly browned at the edges
5. Remove from heat and divide turkey between 4 plates
6. Add the spinach to the pan along with ½ cup of water and steam, stirring frequently for about 2 mins. Remove the greens and lemons with tongs or a slotted spoon and divide between plates
7. Serve topped with dried thyme

Nutrition:

- Calories 204
- Fat 8g
- Carbs 8g
- Fiber 4g
- Protein 30g

Chili Chicken Curry

Prep Time: 5 mins

Servings: 4

Cooking: 20 mins

Ingredients:

- 14 oz kidney beans
- 3 tbsp red curry paste
- 1 lb. ground chicken
- 1 tbsp tomato paste
- 12 oz black beans
- 1 tbsp chili powder
- 2 tsp dried oregano
- 1 cup tomato sauce
- Vegetable oil

Directions:

1. Heat the oil in a rice cooker
2. Add curry paste and stir

3. Place the chicken into a heated rice cooker
4. Cook until cooked thoroughly
5. Once cooked add the beans, tomato paste, and sauce.

Nutrition:

- Calories 315
- Protein 39g
- Carbs 25g
- Fat 9g

Saucy Chicken

Prep Time: 15 mins

Servings: 4

Cooking: 10 mins

Ingredients:

- 8 chicken tights
- 1 cup chicken broth
- 1 tbsp sherry vinegar
- 1½ cup roasted red peppers, chopped
- 4 crushed garlic cloves
- 1½ cup diced russet potatoes
- 2 tsp chopped thyme leaves

Directions:

1. Preheat oven to 425F
2. Heat olive oil in a pan over medium-high heat
3. Season the chicken tights with salt and pepper and place into heated oil, skin side down

4. Cook the chicken without moving around for 3 mins or until browned
5. Transfer to a plate and repeat with remaining chicken
6. Add the garlic and thyme to the same skillet. Cook until fragrant.
7. Add the potatoes, chicken broth, red peppers, and vinegar to the pan
8. Bring to boil and once boils remove from the heat
9. Return the chicken to the pan, skin side up and place in the oven
10. Braise the chicken for 30 mins or until the potatoes are tender

Nutrition:

- Calories 125
- Protein 17g
- Carbs 17g
- Fat 6g

Chicken Fried Rice

Prep Time: 6 mins

Servings: 2

Cooking: 8 mins

Ingredients:

- 2 tbsp Oil
- 2 minced garlic cloves
- 4 oz cubed chicken breast
- 4 oz Shrimp
- 1 cup Mix vegetables-frozen
- 12 oz Overnight rice
- 1 tbsp Fish Sauce
- 1 tbsp Soy Sauce
- ¼ tsp Oyster Sauce
- ¼ tsp White Pepper
- 2 Eggs

Directions:

1. In a pan, add oil and garlic, cook, until the aroma of the garlic becomes present
2. Add shrimp, chicken, and vegetables
3. Put in in rice and stir to combine with veggies
4. Add soy sauce, fish sauce, oyster sauce, salt, and pepper and stir the rice for a few mins
5. Use a spatula to make a gap in the center of the rice
6. Dispense eggs in the center and let it sit for 30 seconds. Use rice to cover eggs and stir as egg cooks.
7. Add some salt and stir a bit more then serve.

Nutrition:

- Calories 306
- Protein 15g
- Carbs 50g
- Fat 5g

Mexican Chicken

Prep Time: 10 mins

Servings: 4

Cooking: 7 hours

Ingredients:

- 4 chicken breasts, skinless and boneless
- ½ cup water
- 16 oz chunky salsa
- 1 and ½ tbsp parsley, chopped
- 1 tsp garlic powder
- ½ tbsp cilantro, chopped
- 1 tsp onion powder
- ½ tbsp oregano, dried
- ½ tsp sweet paprika
- 1 tsp chili powder
- ½ tsp cumin, ground

Directions:

1. Put the water in your slow cooker, add chicken breasts, salsa, parsley, garlic powder, cilantro, onion powder, oregano, paprika, chili powder, cumin and black pepper to the taste, toss, cover and cook on Low for 7 hours.
2. Divide the whole mix between plates and serve.

Nutrition:

- Calories 200
- Fat 4g
- Fiber 2g
- Carbs 12g
- Protein 9g

Chicken Breast Stew

Prep Time: 10 mins

Servings: 4

Cooking: 8 hours

Ingredients:

- 1 yellow onion, chopped
- 2 lbs chicken breasts, skinless and boneless
- 4 oz canned jalapenos, drained and chopped
- 1 green bell pepper, chopped
- 4 oz canned green chilies, drained and chopped
- 7 oz tomato sauce
- 14 oz canned tomatoes, chopped
- 2 tbsp coconut oil, melted
- 3 garlic cloves, minced
- 1 tbsp chili powder
- 1 tbsp cumin, ground
- 2 tsp oregano, dried
- A bunch of cilantro, chopped

- 1 avocado, pitted, peeled and sliced

Directions:

1. Grease the slow cooker with the melted oil, add onion, chicken, jalapenos, bell pepper, green chilies, tomato sauce, tomatoes, garlic, chili powder, cumin, oregano and black pepper, stir, cover and cook on Low for 8 hours.
2. Add cilantro, shred chicken breasts using 2 forks, stir the stew, divide into bowls and top with avocado slices.

Nutrition:

- Calories 205
- Fat 4g
- Fiber 5g
- Carbs 9g
- Protein 11g

Vegetable Chicken Enchiladas

Prep Time: 10 mins

Servings: 4

Cooking: 40 mins

Ingredients:

- nonstick cooking spray
- 1 large onion, peeled and chopped
- 1 green bell pepper, seeded and chopped
- 1 large zucchini, chopped
- 1 cup cooked, chopped chicken breast
- 3/4 cup red enchilada sauce
- 2 (8-ounce) cans no salt added tomato sauce
- 8 (6-inch) corn tortillas
- 2/3 cup shredded reduced fat Monterey Jack cheese

Directions:

1. Preheat oven to 375°F.

2. Spray large skillet with nonstick cooking spray. Sauté onion for 5 mins, stirring occasionally. Add bell pepper and zucchini; cook for 5 mins more. Stir in chicken; set aside.

3. Meanwhile, combine enchilada sauce and tomato sauce in a small bowl; add 1/2 cup to vegetable and chicken mixture.

4. Soften tortillas on the stovetop or in the microwave. Dip each tortilla in sauce and place equal amounts of vegetable and chicken mixture on one side. Roll up and place in a 13x9-inch baking pan. Pour remaining sauce over the top.

5. Cover loosely with foil and bake for 20 to 25 mins. Remove cover and sprinkle cheese over top; bake for 5 mins more. Serve while hot.

Nutrition:

- Calories 311
- Carbs 41 g
- Fiber 7 g
- Protein 22 g
- Fat 8 g

Turkey Meatloaf

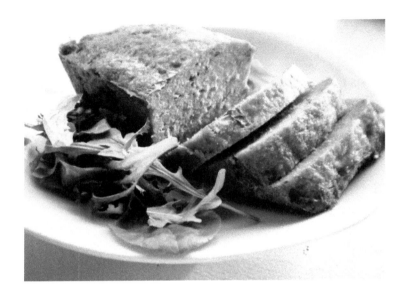

Prep Time: 5 mins

Servings: 5

Cooking: 25 mins

Ingredients:

- 1 lb lean ground turkey
- 1/2 cup regular oats, dry

- 1 large egg, whole
- 1 tbsp onion, dehydrated flakes
- 1/4 cup ketchup*

Directions:

1. Combine all ingredients and mix well.
2. Bake in a loaf pan at 350 °F for 25 mins or to an internal temperature of 165 °F.
3. Cut into five slices and serve.

Nutrition:

- Calories 191
- Fat 7 g
- Protein 23 g
- Carbs 9 g
- Fiber 1 g

Shepherd's Pie

Prep Time: 15 mins

Servings: 4

Cooking: 40 mins

Ingredients:

For potatoes

- 1 lb Russet potatoes (or other white baking potatoes), rinsed, peeled, and cubed into 1/2-inch to 3/4-inch pieces
- 1/4 cup low-fat plain yogurt (or low-fat sour cream)
- 1 cup fat-free milk, hot
- 1/4 tsp ground black pepper
- 1 tbsp fresh chives, rinsed, dried, and chopped (or 1 tsp dried)

For filling

- 4 cups mixed cooked vegetables—such as carrots, celery, onions, bell peppers, mushrooms, or peas (or a 1-lb bag frozen mixed vegetables)
- 2 cups low-sodium chicken broth
- 1 cup quick-cooking oats
- 1 cup grilled or roasted chicken breast, diced (about 2 small breasts)
- 1 tbsp fresh parsley, rinsed, dried, and chopped (or 1 tsp dried)
- 1/4 tsp ground black pepper
- Nonstick cooking spray

Directions:

1. Place potatoes in a medium saucepan, and add enough cold water to cover by 1 inch. Bring to a boil (about 20 to 30 mins)
2. In the meanwhile combine the vegetables, chicken broth, and oats in a medium saucepan. Bring to a boil (about 5–7 mins) Add chicken, and continue to simmer until heated through. Season with parsley and pepper.
3. When potatoes have about 5 mins left to cook, preheat the oven to 450°F.

4. When the potatoes are done, drain and dry them well, then mash with a potato masher or big fork.

5. Add the yogurt, hot milk, and salt. Stir well until smooth. Season with pepper and chives.

6. Lightly spray an 8- by 8-inch square baking dish, or four individual 4-inch ceramic bowls, with cooking spray. Place filling in the bottom of prepared dish (about 2 cups each for individual bowls). Carefully spread potato mixture on top of the chicken and vegetables (about 1 cup each for individual bowls) so they remain in two separate layers.

7. Bake in the preheated oven for about 10 mins, or until the potatoes are browned and chicken is reheated (to a minimum internal temperature of 165°F). Serve immediately.

Nutrition:

- Calories 336

- Fat 4 g

- Fiber 7 g

- Protein 24 g

- Carbs 54 g

Turkey Breast and Sweet Potato Mix

Prep Time: 10 mins

Servings: 4

Cooking : 8 hours

Ingredients:

- 3 sweet potatoes, cut into wedges
- 1 cup dried cherries, pitted
- 2 white onions, cut into wedges
- 1/3 cup water
- 1 tsp onion powder
- 1 tsp garlic powder
- 1 tsp parsley flakes
- 1 tsp thyme, dried
- 1 tsp sage, dried
- 1 tsp paprika, dried

Directions:

1. Put the turkey breast in your slow cooker, add sweet potatoes, cherries, onions, water, parsley, garlic and onion powder, thyme, sage, paprika and pepper, toss, cover and cook on Low for 8 hours.
2. Discard bone from turkey breast, slice meat and divide between plates.
3. Serve with the veggies and the cherries on the side.

Nutrition:

- Calories 220
- Fat 5g
- Fiber 4g
- Carbs 8g
- Protein 15g

Italian Chicken

Prep Time: 10 mins

Servings: 4

Cooking: 5 hours

Ingredients:

- 4 chicken breasts, skinless and boneless
- 6 Italian sausages, sliced
- 5 garlic cloves, minced
- 1 white onion, chopped
- 1 tsp Italian seasoning
- A drizzle of olive oil
- 1 tsp garlic powder
- 29 oz canned tomatoes, chopped
- 15 oz tomato sauce, no-salt-added
- 1 cup water
- ½ cup balsamic vinegar

Directions:

1. Put chicken and sausage slices in your slow cooker, add garlic, onion, Italian seasoning, the oil, tomatoes, tomato sauce, garlic powder, water and the vinegar, cover and cook on High for 5 hours.
2. Stir chicken and sausage mix, divide between plates and serve.

Nutrition:

- Calories 237
- Fat 4g
- Fiber 3g
- Carbs 12g
- Protein 13g

Chicken Breast and Cinnamon Veggie Mix

Prep Time: 10 mins

Servings: 4

Cooking: 6 hours

Ingredients:

- 2 red bell peppers, chopped
- 2 lbs chicken breasts, skinless and boneless
- 4 garlic cloves, minced
- 1 yellow onion, chopped
- 2 tsps paprika
- 1 cup low sodium chicken stock
- 2 tsps cinnamon powder
- ¼ tsp nutmeg, ground

Directions:

In a bowl, mix bell peppers with chicken breasts, garlic, onion, paprika, cinnamon and nutmeg, toss to coat, transfer everything to your slow cooker, add stock, cover, cook on Low for 6 hours, divide everything between plates and serve.

Nutrition:

Calories 200

Fat 3g

Fiber 5g

Carbs 13g

Protein 8g

Buffalo & Ranch Chicken Meatloaf

Prep Time: 10 mins

Servings: 6

Cooking: 35 mins

Ingredients:

- ½ cup ranch dressing
- ¼ cup buffalo wing sauce
- 675g ground chicken
- 120g chicken stuffing mix
- ½ cup feta cheese
- 1 sliced celery stalk
- 2 chopped green onion
- 1 egg

Directions:

1. Preheat oven to 375 degrees and lightly grease a 6 x 4-inch loaf tin with olive oil

2. Mix all your egg and dry Ingredients, along with half of your dressing ingredients: together until fully incorporated using your hands

3. Once combined, add your meat mixture into your greased loaf tin, top with the other half of your dressing ingredients: and set to bake until done (about 30 to 35 mins)

4. Tip: Use a thermometer to determine doneness by inserting it into the thickest part of the meatloaf. Ensure it reads 165 F.

Nutrition:

- Calories 119
- Protein 6g
- Carbs 14g
- Fat 4g

Mexican Beef Mix

Prep Time: 10 mins

Servings: 6

Cooking: 8 hours

Ingredients:

- 1 yellow onion, chopped
- 2 tbsp sweet paprika
- 15 oz canned tomatoes, no-salt-added, roasted and chopped
- 1 tsp cumin, ground
- 1 tsp olive oil
- A pinch of nutmeg, ground
- 5 lbs beef roast
- Juice of 1 lemon
- ¼ cup apple cider vinegar

Directions:

1. Heat up a pan with the oil over medium-high heat, add onions, stir, brown them for 2-3 mins, transfer them to your slow cooker, add paprika, tomato, cumin, nutmeg, lemon juice, vinegar, black pepper and beef, toss to coat, cover and cook on Low for 8 hours.
2. Slice roast, divide between plates and serve with tomatoes and onions mix on the side.

Nutrition:

- Calories 250
- Fat 5g
- Fiber 2g
- Carbs 8g
- Protein 15g

Maple Beef Tenderloin

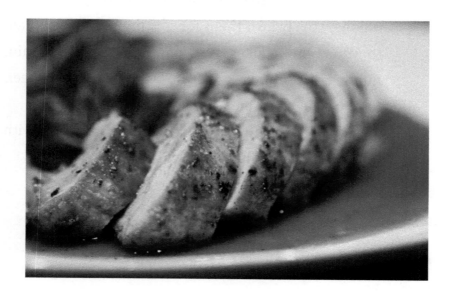

Prep Time: 10 mins

Servings: 4

Cooking: 8 hours

Ingredients:

- A pinch of nutmeg, ground
- 2 lbs beef tenderloin, trimmed

- 4 apples, cored and sliced
- 2 tbsp maple syrup

Directions:

1. Place half of the apples in your slow cooker, sprinkle the nutmeg over them, add beef tenderloin, top with the rest of the apples, drizzle the maple syrup, cover and cook on Low for 8 hours.
2. Slice beef tenderloin, divide between plates and serve with apple slices and cooking juices on top.

Nutrition:

- Calories 240
- Fat 4g
- Fiber 5g
- Carbs 14g
- Protein 14 g

Beef and Cabbage Stew

Prep Time: 10 mins

Servings: 6

Cooking: 8 hours

Ingredients:

- 1 tbsp olive oil
- 2 lbs beef loin, cubed
- 3 garlic cloves, minced
- 6 baby carrots, halved
- 2 onions, chopped
- Black pepper to the taste
- 1 cabbage head, shredded
- 3 cups veggie stock
- 28 oz canned tomatoes, no-salt-added, drained and chopped
- 3 big sweet potatoes, cubed

Directions:

Heat up a pan with the oil over medium-high heat, add meat, brown for a few mins on each side, transfer to your slow cooker, add black pepper, carrots, garlic, onion, potatoes, cabbage, stock and tomatoes, stir well, cover, cook on Low for 8 hours, divide the stew into bowls and serve right away.

Nutrition:

- Calories 270
- Fat 5g
- Fiber 4g
- Carbs 14g
- Protein 7g

Greek Beef

Prep Time: 1 day

Servings: 6

Cooking: 8 hours

Ingredients:

- 3 lbs beeg shoulder, boneless
- ¼ cup olive oil
- 2 tsps oregano, dried
- ¼ cup lemon juice
- 2 tsps mustard
- 2 tsps mint
- 6 garlic cloves, minced

Directions:

1. In a bowl, mix oil with lemon juice, oregano, mint, mustard, garlic and pepper, whisk, rub the meat with the marinade, cover and keep in the fridge for 1 day.

2. Transfer to your slow cooker along with the marinade, cover, cook on Low for 8 hours, slice the roast and serve.

Nutrition:

- Calories 260
- Fat 4g
- Fiber 6g
- Carbs 14g
- Protein 8 g

Roast and Veggies

Prep Time: 10 mins

Servings: 6

Cooking: 4 hours

Ingredients:

- 1 lb sweet potatoes, chopped
- 3 and ½ lbs beef roast, trimmed
- 8 medium carrots, chopped
- 15 oz canned tomatoes, no-salt-added and chopped
- 1 yellow onion, chopped
- Zest of 1 lemon, grated
- Juice of 1 lemon
- 4 garlic cloves, minced
- Black pepper to the taste
- ½ cup kalamata olives, pitted

Directions:

1. Put potatoes in your slow cooker, carrots, tomatoes, onions, lemon juice and zest, beef, black pepper and garlic, stir, cover and cook on High for 4 hours.
2. Transfer meat to a cutting board, slice it and divide between plates.
3. Transfer the veggies to a bowl, mash, mix them with olives, and add next to the meat.

Nutrition:

- Calories 250
- Fat 4g
- Fiber 3g
- Carbs 15g
- Protein 13g

Pork Medallions

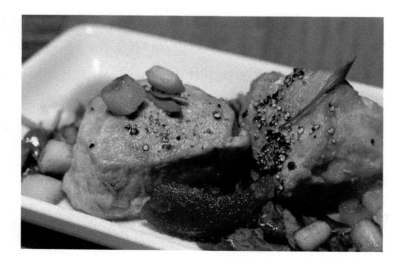

Prep Time: 10 mins

Servings: 4

Cooking: 20 mins

Ingredients:

- 1 lb pork tenderloin, trimmed and cut into 1-inch-thick slices
- 2 tsps minced garlic

- 1 tsp dried rosemary
- 1½ tbsp olive oil, divided
- 1 cup low-sodium chicken stock
- 1 cup carrots, halved and thinly sliced
- 3 tbsp water
- ½ tsp freshly ground black pepper
- 2 cups frozen lima beans, thawed
- 1 cup frozen spinach, thawed

Directions:

1. Gently divide pork slices to ½-inch-thick medallions with a meat mallet or the heel of your hand.
2. Combine garlic and rosemary in a small bowl.
3. Heat a large skillet over medium heat. Add 1 tbsp of olive oil and swirl to coat. Add the pork to the pan and cook for 4 mins without turning. Turn and cook for 3 mins or until done. Remove pork from pan and keep warm.
4. Add garlic mixture; sauté for 1 minute or until fragrant. Add chicken stock and cook for 30 seconds or until reduced to ½ cup. Remove pan from heat.
5. Heat a second large nonstick skillet over medium heat. Add remaining olive oil and swirl to coat. Add carrots and cook for 2 mins. Stir in water and black pepper. Cover and cook for 2 mins until carrots are crisp

tender. Stir in lima beans and spinach, Cook for 3 mins or until thoroughly heated.

6. Divide vegetable mixture among 4 plates. Top each serving with pork and sauce.

Nutrition:

- Calories 317
- Fat 11g
- Carbs 28g
- Fiber 8g
- Protein 28g

Pork Salad with Walnuts and Peaches

Prep Time: 15 mins

Servings: 4

Cooking: 10 mins

Ingredients:

- 1 tbsp olive oil
- 1 lb pork tenderloin, cut into 1-in ch cubes
- 1 (10-ounce) bag fresh spinach leaves
- 1 peach, pitted and sliced
- ¼ cup walnuts
- Balsamic vinegar

Directions:

1. Heat the olive oil in a large nonstick skillet over medium-high heat. Add the pork and cook until it is browned on the outside and cooked through (3 to 4 mins per side). Remove from heat and set aside.

2. Make a bed of spinach on each individual serving plate. Arrange peach slices over the spinach. Top with the cooked pork and sprinkle with walnuts. Drizzle balsamic vinegar over the salad.

3. Enjoy immediately.

Nutrition:

- Calories 230
- Fat 14g
- Carbs 6g
- Protein 21g

Pork, White Bean, and Spinach Soup

Prep Time: 10 mins

Servings: 4

Cooking: 15 mins

Ingredients:

- 1 tbsp olive oil
- 8 oz pork tenderloin or boneless pork chops, cut into 1-inch cubes
- 4 garlic cloves, minced
- 2 tsps paprika
- 1 (14.5-ounce) can diced salt-free tomatoes
- 4 cups low-sodium chicken broth
- 1 bunch spinach, ribs removed and chopped, about 8 cups, lightly packed
- 2 (15-ounce) cans white beans, drained and rinsed

Directions:

1. Heat the oil in a Dutch oven or heavy-bottom pot over medium-high heat. Season pork with a pinch of salt. When the pan is hot, add pork and cook, stirring occasionally, for about 2 mins, or long enough to encourage a good sear and brown sides. Transfer to a plate.

2. In the same pot, add the garlic and paprika. Cook, stirring often, until fragrant (about 30 seconds). Add tomatoes and increase heat to high and stir to scrape down any browned bits. Add broth and bring to a boil.

3. Add spinach until it just wilts (about 2 to 3 mins).

Nutrition:

- Calories 327
- Fat 8g
- Carbs 41g
- Protein 26g

Orange-Beef Stir-Fry

Prep Time: 10 mins

Servings: 2

Cooking: 10 mins

Ingredients:

- 1 tbsp cornstarch
- ¼ cup cold water
- ¼ cup orange juice
- 1 tbsp reduced-sodium soy sauce
- ½ lb boneless beef sirloin steak, cut into thin strips
- 2 tsps olive oil, divided
- 3 cups frozen stir-fry vegetable blend
- 1 garlic clove, minced

Directions:

1. In a small bowl, combine cornstarch, cold water, orange juice, and soy sauce until smooth and set aside

2. In a large skillet or wok, stir-fry beef in 1 tsp of olive oil for 3 to 4 mins or until no longer pink
3. Remove with a slotted spoon and keep warm
4. Stir-fry the vegetable blend and garlic in the remaining oil for 3 mins. Stir cornstarch mixture and add to the pan. Bring to a boil
5. Cook stirring constantly, for 2 mins or until thickened. Add the beef and heat through.

Nutrition:

- Calories 268
- Fat 10g, Carbs 8g
- Fiber 3g
- Protein 26g

Quick Chicken Fajitas

Prep Time: 10 mins

Servings: 4

Cooking: 15 mins

Ingredients:

- Cooking spray
- 4 cups frozen bell pepper strips
- 2 cups onion, sliced
- 1 tsp ground cumin
- 1 tsp chili powder
- 2 (10-ounce) cans no-salt diced tomatoes and green chilies (Ro-Tel brand)
- 8 (6-inch) whole-wheat flour tortillas, warmed

Directions:

1. Spray a large skillet with cooking spray. Preheat skillet to medium-high heat. Add the bell peppers and onions

and cook for 7 mins or until tender, stirring occasionally. Remove from skillet and set aside

2. Add chicken to skillet. Sprinkle with cumin and chili powder. Cook for 4 mins until no longer pink and an instant-read thermometer registers 165°F

3. Return peppers and onions to skillet; add drained tomatoes and green chilies. Cook for 2 mins more or until hot

4. Divide mixture evenly between tortillas and serve immediately.

Nutrition:

- Calories 424
- Fat 8g
- Carbs 51g
- Fiber 26g
- Protein 33g

Roasted Turkey

Prep Time: 15 mins

Servings: 6

Cooking: 45 mins

Ingredients:

- 1 whole turkey
- 2 tsp garlic paste
- 1 tsp ginger powder
- 2 tbsp soya sauce
- 1 tsp cayenne pepper
- 3 tbsp lemon juice
- 2 tbsp red wine vinegar
- ½ tsp mustard powder
- 1 tsp cinnamon powder
- 2 tbsp sesame seeds oil

Directions:

1. In a bowl add garlic paste, ginger powder, cayenne pepper, black pepper, cinnamon powder, mustard powder, lemon juice, oil, vinegar, soya sauce and salt, mix well
2. Now pour this marinate over turkey and rub with hands all over it
3. Cover and leave to marinade for 15-20 mins
4. Preheat oven at 355 degrees
5. Spread aluminum foil in baking tray and place turkey on it
6. Bake for 40-45 mins or till nicely golden.

Nutrition:

- Calories 244
- Fat 7g
- Protein 44g
- Carbs 3g

Honey Garlic Chicken Drumsticks

Prep Time: 25 mins

Servings: 6

Cooking: 35 mins

Ingredients:

- 8 chicken drumsticks
- 3 tsp garlic powder
- 1 tsp ginger powder
- 3 tbsp soya sauce
- 1 tsp cayenne pepper
- 2 tbsp Barbecue sauce
- 2 tbsp lime juice
- ¼ cup apple cider vinegar
- 2 tbsp olive oil
- 3 tbsp honey

Directions:

1. In a bowl add ginger powder, garlic powder, soya sauce, honey, vinegar, lime juice, barbecue sauce, salt, pepper and toss to combine
2. Add in chicken drumsticks and mix well, leave to marinade for 20 mins. Preheat oven at 355F
3. Transfer drumsticks in baking tray and bake for 30-35 mins or till golden brown

Nutrition:

- Calories 122
- Protein 1g
- Carbs 15g
- Fat 3g

Southwestern Chicken and Pasta

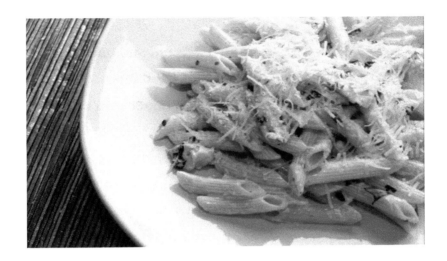

Prep Time: 10 mins

Servings: 2

Cooking: 10 mins

Ingredients:

- 1 cup uncooked whole-wheat rigatoni
- 2 boneless, skinless chicken breasts, 4 oz each, cut into cubes

- 1/4 cup salsa

Directions:

1. Fill a pot with water up to ¾ full and boil it
2. Add pasta to water and cook until it is al dente
3. Drain the pasta while rinsing under cold water
4. Preheat a skillet with cooking oil, then cook the chicken for 10 mins until golden on both sides.
5. Add tomato sauce, salsa, cumin, garlic powder, black beans, corn, and chili powder.
6. Stir while cooking the mixture for a few mins. Add in pasta.
7. Serve with 2 tbsp cheese on top.

Nutrition:

- Calories 245
- Fat 16.3 g
- Carbs 19.3g
- Protein 33.3 g

Chicken Sliders

Prep Time: 10 mins

Servings: 4

Cooking: 10 mins

Ingredients:

- 10 oz ground chicken breast
- 1 tbsp black pepper
- 1 tbsp minced garlic
- 1 tbsp balsamic vinegar
- 1/2 cup minced onion
- 1 fresh chili pepper, minced
- 1 tbsp fennel seed, crushed
- 4 whole-wheat mini buns
- 4 lettuce leaves
- 4 tomato slices

Directions:

1. Combine all the ingredients: except the wheat buns, tomato, and lettuce.
2. Mix well and refrigerate the mixture for 1 hour.
3. Divide the mixture into 4 patties.
4. Broil the patties on a greased baking sheet until golden brown.
5. Place the chicken patties in the whole wheat buns along with lettuce and tomato.

Nutrition:

- Calories 224
- Fat 4.5 g
- Carbs 10.2 g
- Protein 67.4 g

Buffalo Chicken Salad Wrap

Prep Time: 10 mins

Servings: 4

Cooking: 10 mins

Ingredients:

- 3-4 oz chicken breasts
- 2 whole chipotle peppers
- 1/4 cup white wine vinegar
- 1/4 cup low-calorie mayonnaise
- 2 diced stalks celery
- 2 carrots, cut into matchsticks
- 1 small yellow onion, diced (about 1/2 cup)
- 1/2 cup thinly sliced rutabaga or another root vegetable
- 4 oz spinach, cut into strips
- 2 whole-grain tortillas (12-inch diameter)

Directions:

1. Set the oven or a grill to heat at 375°F. Bake the chicken for 10 mins per side.
2. Blend chipotle peppers with mayonnaise and wine vinegar in the blender.
3. Dice the baked chicken into cubes or small chunks.
4. Mix the chipotle mixture with all the ingredients: except tortillas and spinach.
5. Spread 2 oz of spinach over tortilla and scoop the stuffing on top.
6. Wrap the tortilla and cut it into the half.

Nutrition:

- Calories 300
- Fat 16.4 g
- Carbs 8.7 g
- Fiber 0.7 g
- Protein 38.5 g

White Chicken Chili

Prep Time: 10 mins

Servings: 8

Cooking: 15 mins

Ingredients:

- 3 tbsp chopped cilantro
- 8 tbsp shredded Monterey jack cheese
- 1 tsp cayenne pepper
- 1 tsp dried oregano
- 1 tsp ground cumin
- 2 tsp chili powder
- 2 minced garlic cloves
- 1 sliced red pepper
- ½ sliced green pepper
- 4 cup low-sodium chicken broth
- 1 can diced tomatoes
- 2 cans white beans
- 1 can white chunk chicken

Directions:

1. Place the chicken broth, tomatoes, and chicken in a large cooking pot
2. Bring the mixture to a boil and then cover it to let it simmer
3. While the mixture is simmering, take a nonstick frying pan, cover it in cooking spray, and add the garlic, peppers, and onions
4. Fry the vegetables until golden brown or to your liking
5. Add the contents of the frying pan to the cooking pot
6. Add the cayenne pepper, oregano, cumin, and chili powder and cover the mixture again
7. Raise the heat up to medium and let it simmer for about 10 more mins
8. Ladle the chili into bowls and serve immediately.

Nutrition:

- Calories 212
- Fat 4g
- Carbs 25g
- Protein 19g

Turkey Club Burger

Prep Time: 10 mins

Servings: 4

Cooking: 15 mins

Ingredients:

For turkey burger

- 12 oz 99 percent fat-free ground turkey
- 1/2 cup scallions (green onions), rinsed and sliced
- 1/4 tsp ground black pepper
- 1 large egg
- 1 tbsp olive oil

For spread

- 2 tbsp light mayonnaise
- 1 tbsp Dijon mustard
- For toppings
- 4 oz spinach or arugula, rinsed and dried
- 4 oz portabella mushroom, rinsed, grilled or broiled, and sliced (optional)

- 4 whole-wheat hamburger buns

Directions:

1. Preheat oven broiler on high temperature (with the rack 3 inches from heat source) or grill on medium-high heat.
2. To prepare burgers, combine ground turkey, scallions, pepper, and egg, and mix well. Form into 1/2- to 3/4-inch thick patties, and coat each lightly with olive oil.
3. Broil or grill burgers for about 7–9 mins on each side (to a minimum internal temperature of 160 °F).
4. Combine mayonnaise and mustard to make a spread.
5. Assemble 3/4 tbsp spread, 1 ounce spinach or arugula, several slices of grilled portabella mushroom (optional), and one burger on each bun.

Nutrition Information:

- Calories 299
- Fat 11 g
- Protein 29 g
- Carbs 26 g

Mango Chicken Stir-Fry

Prep Time: 10 mins

Servings: 4

Cooking: 15 mins

Ingredients:

- nonstick cooking spray
- 1 lb boneless, skinless chicken breasts, cut into bite-size chunks
- 1/4 cup pineapple juice
- 3 tbsp low-sodium soy sauce
- 1/4 tsp ground ginger
- 1 red bell pepper, cut into bite-size strips
- 2 mangos, pitted and cut into bite-size strips
- 1/4 cup toasted, slivered almonds ground black pepper to taste
- 2 cups cooked brown rice

Directions:

1. Spray a large wok or skillet with nonstick cooking spray.
2. Sauté chicken over medium-high heat until cooked through, about 10 mins.
3. In a small bowl, stir together pineapple juice, soy sauce, and ginger. Add sauce and bell pepper to the skillet.
4. Cook and stir for about 5 mins until peppers are crisp-tender.
5. Add the mango and almonds to the wok or skillet and cook until hot. Season with ground black pepper to taste.
6. Serve each cup of stir-fry over 1/2 cup of brown rice.

Nutrition:

- Calories 387
- Carbs 47 g
- Protein 31 g
- Fat 9 g

Chicken Couscous

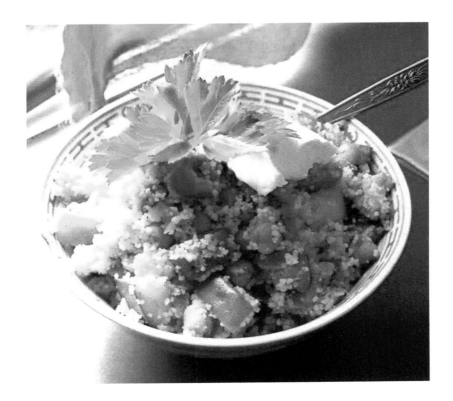

Prep Time: 5 mins

Servings: 4

Cooking: 30 mins

Ingredients:

- 1 tbsp olive oil
- 1 lb skinless chicken legs, split (about 4 whole legs)
- 1 tbsp Moroccan spice blend*
- 1 cup carrots, rinsed, peeled, and diced
- 1 cup onion, diced
- 1/4 cup lemon juice
- 2 cups low-sodium chicken broth
- 1/2 cup ripe black olives, sliced
- 1 tbsp chili sauce (optional)

For couscous

- 1 cup low-sodium chicken broth
- 1 cup couscous (try whole-wheat couscous)
- 1 tbsp fresh mint, rinsed, dried, and shredded thin (or 1 tsp dried)

Directions:

1. Heat olive oil in a large sauté pan. Add chicken legs, and brown on all sides, about 2–3 mins per side. Remove chicken from pan and put on a plate with a cover to hold warm.
2. Add spice blend to sauté pan and toast gently.

3. Add carrots and onion to sauté pan, and cook for about 3–4 mins or until the onions have turned clear, but not brown.

4. Add lemon juice, chicken broth, and olives to sauté pan, and bring to a boil over high heat. Add chicken legs, and return to a boil. Cover and gently simmer for about 10–15 mins (to a minimum internal temperature of 165 °F).

5. Meanwhile, prepare the couscous by bringing chicken broth to a boil in a saucepan. Add couscous and remove from the heat. Cover and let stand for 10 mins.

6. Fluff couscous with a fork, and gently mix in the mint.

7. When chicken is cooked, add salt. Serve two chicken legs over 1/2 cup couscous topped with 1/2 cup sauce in a serving bowl. Add chili sauce to taste.

Nutrition:

- Calories 333
- Fat 12 g
- Protein 24 g
- Carbs 36 g

Exotic Jerk Chicken

Prep Time: 8 mins

Servings: 10

Cooking: 1 hour

Ingredients:

- 1/2 tsp cinnamon, ground
- 1-1/2 tsp allspice, ground
- 1-1/2 tsp black pepper, ground
- 1 tsp hot pepper, crushed, dried
- 2 tsp oregano, crushed
- 2 tsp thyme, crushed
- 6 cloves garlic, finely chopped
- 1 cup onion, pureed or finely chopped
- 1/4 cup vinegar
- 3 tbsp brown sugar
- 8 pieces chicken, skinless (4 breasts, 4 drumsticks)

Directions:

1. Preheat oven to 350 degrees F. Wash chicken and pat dry. Combine all ingredients: except chicken in large bowl. Rub seasonings over chicken and marinate in refrigerator for 6 hours or longer.
2. Space chicken evenly on nonstick or lightly greased baking pan.
3. Cover with aluminum foil and bake for 40 mins. Remove foil and continue baking for an additional 30– 40 mins or until the meat can easily be pulled away from the bone with a fork.

Nutrition:

*   Calories 113
*   Fat 3 g
*   Fiber 1 g
*   Protein 16 g
*   Carbs 6 g

Chicken Vegetable Creole

Prep Time: 8 mins

Servings: 6

Cooking: 20 mins

Ingredients:

- nonstick cooking spray
- 1 lb boneless, skinless chicken breasts, cut into large chunks
- 1 large onion, chopped
- 1 (14-1/2-ounce) can diced tomatoes
- 1/3 cup tomato paste
- 2 stalks celery, chopped
- 1-1/2 tsp garlic powder
- 1 tsp onion powder
- 1/4 tsp red pepper flakes
- 1/8 tsp ground black pepper
- 1-1/2 cups broccoli florets

Directions:

1. Spray a large skillet with nonstick cooking spray and heat over medium heat.
2. Add chicken and onion; cook, stirring frequently, for 10 mins.
3. Stir in all remaining ingredients: except broccoli and cook for 5 mins, stirring occasionally.
4. Stir in broccoli, cook for 5 mins more. Serve while hot.

Nutrition:

- Calories 143
- Carbs 11 g
- Protein 19 g
- Fat 3 g

Crispy Oven-Fried Chicken

Prep Time: 5 mins

Servings: 4

Cooking: 1 hour

Ingredients:

- 1/2 cup fat-free milk or buttermilk
- 1 tsp poultry seasoning
- 1 cup cornflakes, crumbled
- 1-1/2 tbsp onion powder
- 1-1/2 tbsp garlic powder
- 2 tsp black pepper
- 2 tsp dried hot pepper, crushed
- 1 tsp ginger, ground
- 8 pieces chicken, skinless (4 breasts, 4 drumsticks)
- a few shakes paprika
- 1 tsp vegetable oil

Directions:

1. Preheat oven to 350 ° F.
2. Add 1/2 tsp of poultry seasoning to milk.
3. Combine all other spices with cornflake crumbs, and place in plastic bag.
4. Wash chicken and pat dry. Dip chicken into milk and shake to remove excess. Quickly shake in bag with seasonings and crumbs, and remove the chicken from the bag.
5. Refrigerate chicken for 1 hour.
6. Remove chicken from refrigerator and sprinkle lightly with paprika for color.
7. Space chicken evenly on greased baking pan.
8. Cover with aluminum foil and bake for 40 mins. Remove foil and continue baking for another 30–40 mins or until meat can easily be pulled away from the bone with fork. Drumsticks may require less baking time than breasts. Crumbs will form crispy "skin."

Nutrition:

- Calories 117
- Fat 3 g
- Protein 17 g
- Carbs 6 g

Turkey Stir-Fry

Prep Time: 5 mins

Servings: 4

Cooking: 12 mins

Ingredients:

- 1 chicken bouillon cube
- 1/2 cup hot water
- 2 tbsp soy sauce
- 1 tbsp cornstarch
- 2 tbsp vegetable oil
- 1/2 tsp garlic powder
- 1 lb turkey, cubed
- 1-3/4 cups carrots, thinly sliced
- 1 cup zucchini, sliced
- 1/2 cup onions, thinly sliced
- 1/4 cup hot water

Directions:

1. Combine chicken bouillon cube and hot water to make broth; stir until dissolved. Combine broth, soy sauce, and cornstarch in small bowl. Set aside

2. Heat oil in skillet over high heat. Add garlic and turkey. Cook, stirring, until turkey is thoroughly cooked and no longer pink in color.

3. Add carrots, zucchini, onion, and water to cooked turkey. Cover and cook, stirring occasionally, until vegetables are tender-crisp, about 5 mins. Uncover; bring turkey mixture to boil. Cook until almost all liquid has evaporated.

4. Stir in cornstarch mixture. Bring to boil, stirring constantly until thickened.

Nutrition:

- Calories 195
- Total Fat 9 g
- Carbs 47 g
- Protein 31 g

Chicken and Broccoli Stir-Fry

Prep Time: 10 mins

Servings: 4

Cooking: 15 mins

Ingredients:

- 2 tbsp sesame oil (or olive oil), divided
- 3 tbsp balsamic vinegar, divided
- 2 tsps ground ginger

Directions:

1. Heat ½ tbsp of olive oil in a wok or large sauté pan over medium heat. Add the cubed chicken and cook until lightly browned and cooked through (about 5 to 7 mins). Transfer chicken to a bowl, cover, and set aside

2. Add 1½ tbsp of olive oil to the pan, along with the garlic and carrots. Cook until the carrots begin to soften (about 3 to 4 mins). Add the thawed broccoli

florets and water chestnuts along with 1 tbsp of balsamic vinegar and cook for 3 to 4 mins

3. Add the remaining balsamic vinegar and ground ginger. Add the cooked chicken and stir until well combined

Nutrition:

- Calories 189
- Fat 9g
- Carbs 12g
- Fiber 3g
- Protein 14g

Quick Chicken Fajitas

Prep Time: 10 mins

Servings: 4

Cooking: 15 mins

Ingredients:

- Cooking spray
- 4 cups frozen bell pepper strips
- 2 cups onion, sliced
- 1 tsp ground cumin
- 1 tsp chili powder
- 2 (10-ounce) cans no-salt diced tomatoes and green chilies (Ro-Tel brand)
- 8 (6-inch) whole-wheat flour tortillas, warmed

Directions:

1. Spray a large skillet with cooking spray. Preheat skillet to medium-high heat. Add the bell peppers and onions

and cook for 7 mins or until tender, stirring occasionally. Remove from skillet and set aside

2. Add chicken to skillet. Sprinkle with cumin and chili powder. Cook for 4 mins until no longer pink and an instant-read thermometer registers 165°F

3. Return peppers and onions to skillet; add drained tomatoes and green chilies. Cook for 2 mins more or until hot

4. Divide mixture evenly between tortillas and serve immediately.

Nutrition:

- Calories 424
- Fat 8g
- Carbs 51g
- Fiber 26g
- Protein 33g

Roasted Turkey

Prep Time: 15 mins

Servings: 6

Cooking: 45 mins

Ingredients:

- 1 whole turkey
- 2 tsp garlic paste
- 1 tsp ginger powder
- 2 tbsp soya sauce
- 1 tsp cayenne pepper
- 3 tbsp lemon juice
- 2 tbsp red wine vinegar
- ½ tsp mustard powder
- 1 tsp cinnamon powder
- 2 tbsp sesame seeds oil

Directions:

1. In a bowl add garlic paste, ginger powder, cayenne pepper, black pepper, cinnamon powder, mustard powder, lemon juice, oil, vinegar, soya sauce and salt, mix well
2. Now pour this marinate over turkey and rub with hands all over it
3. Cover and leave to marinade for 15-20 mins
4. Preheat oven at 355 degrees
5. Spread aluminum foil in baking tray and place turkey on it
6. Bake for 40-45 mins or till nicely golden.

Nutrition:

- Calories 244
- Fat 7g
- Protein 44g
- Carbs 3g

Honey Garlic Chicken Drumsticks

Prep Time: 15 mins

Servings: 6

Cooking: 35 mins

Ingredients:

- 8 chicken drumsticks
- 3 tsp garlic powder
- 1 tsp ginger powder
- 3 tbsp soya sauce
- 1 tsp cayenne pepper
- 2 tbsp Barbecue sauce
- 2 tbsp lime juice
- ¼ cup apple cider vinegar
- 2 tbsp olive oil
- 3 tbsp honey

Directions:

1. In a bowl add ginger powder, garlic powder, soya sauce, honey, vinegar, lime juice, barbecue sauce, salt, pepper and toss to combine
2. Add in chicken drumsticks and mix well, leave to marinade for 20 mins. Preheat oven at 355 degrees
3. Transfer drumsticks in baking tray and bake for 30-35 mins or till golden brown

Nutrition:

- Calories 122
- Protein 1g
- Carbs 15g
- Fat 3g

Chicken and Zucchini Pasta

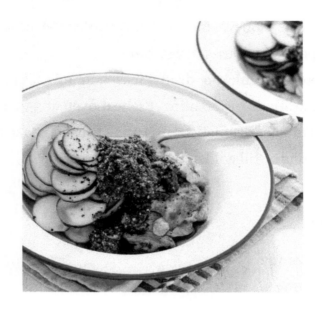

Prep Time: 10 mins

Servings: 2

Cooking: 10 mins

Ingredients:

- 1 cup uncooked whole-wheat pasta

- 2 boneless, skinless chicken breasts, 4 oz each, cut into cubes
- 1cup zucchini chopped
- 1 tsp garlic powder

Directions:

1. Fill a pot with water up to ¾ full and boil it
2. Add pasta to water and cook until it is al dente
3. Drain the pasta while rinsing under cold water
4. Preheat a skillet with cooking oil, then cook the chicken for 10 mins until golden on both sides.
5. Add zucchini and garlic powder.
6. Stir while cooking the mixture for a few mins. Add in pasta.
7. Serve with 2 tbsp cheese on top.

Nutrition:

- Calories 245
- Fat 16.3 g
- Carbs 19.3g
- Protein 33.3 g

Chicken Sliders

Prep Time: 10 mins

Servings: 4

Cooking: 10 mins

Ingredients:

- 10 oz ground chicken breast
- 1 tbsp black pepper
- 1 tbsp minced garlic
- 1 tbsp balsamic vinegar
- 1/2 cup minced onion
- 1 fresh chili pepper, minced
- 1 tbsp fennel seed, crushed
- 4 whole-wheat mini buns
- 4 lettuce leaves
- 4 tomato slices

Directions:

1. Combine all the ingredients: except the wheat buns, tomato, and lettuce.
2. Mix well and refrigerate the mixture for 1 hour.
3. Divide the mixture into 4 patties.
4. Broil the patties on a greased baking sheet until golden brown.
5. Place the chicken patties in the whole wheat buns along with lettuce and tomato.

Nutrition:

- Calories 224
- Fat 4.5 g
- Carbs 10.2 g
- Protein 67.4 g

Lightning Source UK Ltd.
Milton Keynes UK
UKHW020813180621
385734UK00005B/111